# PTSD

## A Spouse's Perspective

# PTSD

## A Spouse's Perspective
## How to survive in a world of PTSD

Erica David

WestBow
PRESS
A DIVISION OF THOMAS NELSON

WestBow Press books may be ordered through booksellers or by contacting:

WestBow Press
A Division of Thomas Nelson
1663 Liberty Drive
Bloomington, IN 47403
www.westbowpress.com
1-(866) 928-1240

Because of the dynamic nature of the Internet, any Web addresses or
links contained in this book may have changed since publication and
may no longer be valid. The views expressed in this work are solely those
of the author and do not necessarily reflect the views of the publisher,
and the publisher hereby disclaims any responsibility for them.

Any people depicted in stock imagery provided by Thinkstock are models,
and such images are being used for illustrative purposes only.

Certain stock imagery © Thinkstock.

ISBN: 978-1-4497-1121-4 (sc)
ISBN: 978-1-4497-1122-1 (e)

Library of Congress Control Number: 2011920322

Printed in the United States of America

WestBow Press rev. date: 1/27/2011

To you, Tim Wampler, my initial therapist.

You are a gentle and caring person who helped me to begin the ascent from the pit of depression and gave me confidence to believe in myself again. Without you, this book would not have been written.

To you, I am eternally grateful.

If PTSD has invaded your world,
you are not alone.

There is hope.

# Contents

# Preface

During my research on PTSD, I consistently found information and research that had been conducted regarding the Veterans that suffer from this illness. However, the issue of PTSD and its effect on the spouse and children has received very little attention in the research arena. I was not able to find one publication that dealt primarily with the effects of PTSD on the spouse and the family of a PTSD Veteran.

Therefore, I decided that I did not want other spouses to endure years of struggling with the unknowns of PTSD as I have. I felt that it was time that one book existed primarily for the spouse that contained information from the definition of PTSD to ways of coping as the caregiver of a person with this illness. It is my desire that this book will help many spouses that are in the same position that I found myself so many years ago.

I have written this book for all the spouses of PTSD sufferers to let you know that 'I understand what you are going through'.

# Acknowledgements

I wish to thank my current therapist and psychiatrist who have walked with me and are continuing to do so as I follow the path to healing. You have been very supportive, encouraging, and have taken the time to talk with me between sessions when life got really tough. You both are wonderful.

To the many new acquaintances and new friends that I have made along the way, you have truly been more than just a shoulder to cry on. For many of you have also endured an abusive past and you can truly say 'I understand'.

To my friend that saw me at my worst and made it a daily ritual to contact me and plan monthly luncheons, thank you. I never had a true friend until I met you.

To my family, I love you.

# Introduction

For so many years as the spouse of someone who has PTSD, I suffered in silence. I assumed the role of family mediator -- trying to prevent my husband from becoming angry and trying to fix the situation if he did. I learned to pick and choose the times I would tell him certain things which usually was after I had rehearsed the conversation repeatedly in my mind and gotten up the courage to reveal the situation.

I always watched my words so as not to cause a scene in public. I wanted others to see his best. In many ways, I assumed the role of his character protector. Not wanting others to be a witness to his anger and irritability.

I do not know the exact date when PTSD slipped into my world. It is as if I woke up one day and realized that PTSD had been secretly occupying space in my home without my permission. It would occasionally cause a scene or an emotional outburst from my husband that seemed out of proportion to the situation. I did not understand why my husband responded in the fashion that he did, but I just thought that was the road our lives had taken.

When my husband returned from the Gulf War, I gradually began to notice changes. As time progressed so did his anger and irritability. He was talkative one minute and withdrawn the next. I never knew which mood would greet me when he came home. I began to think it was my fault. Everything became personal. I began to feel inadequate as his wife and as a person. My husband was different some how, but I could not exactly put into words what I saw. Many days I was not sure that I wanted to continue in this life that had been dealt me.

I began slipping into a black hole. I found myself in a dry land. Each day, it seemed I sank deeper, and I did not know how to get out. The need to escape became a constant companion. When asked, "Where?" I did not know. Just away. "Why?" Maybe to reassess my life hoping that somehow distance would change the feelings that tormented me inside.

I had slipped into survival mode. My doctor kept asking me if I was depressed. I found that question quite humorous as I never thought of myself as someone who could become depressed. But my doctor kept saying there was something about my eyes. After repeatedly seeing the doctor for symptoms that could not result in a diagnosis, I began to wonder if she knew something about me that I did not.

Perhaps it is true that the eyes are the pathway to the soul. For my eyes revealed the sadness I felt inside. I believed that nobody would or could understand and that I could not possibly tell anyone about what I felt. After all, what would they think of me?

I learned to live behind the mask that was always a part of my daily attire. I wanted people to believe that everything was well and that I was happy with no problems. It was easier to live life behind the façade than face people seeking answers to questions that I did not know the answers to myself. All I knew was that inside I was sad. Alone. It seemed the pain was incurable. The sadness turned into withdrawal from people along with a barrage of feelings that I did not understand.

Why not suicide? Certainly the thought was a constant occurrence. Stepping in front of the transfer truck going 70 plus mph would have been easy. But my instinct to live was greater than my desire to die – at least at that moment.

My mind became a conglomeration of major interstates with hundreds of lanes of thoughts traveling at enormous speeds. Lights flashing. Horns blowing. I knew that I needed help before a major collision of my thoughts occurred. Maybe the doctor was right. Depression had invaded my world and forced me into a black bottomless hole. I had to break my fall and find something to hold onto.

Living with a spouse who suffers from PTSD had left me depressed with feelings of insecurity, low self-esteem, and wondering if his mood swings were my fault. I never knew how he would respond to situations which resulted in me quite often walking on egg shells.

Through my husband's counselor, I became aware of a counseling session for the spouses of those veterans attending counseling for PTSD. Reluctantly, I attended the first session.

It was a small group of four ladies and two counselors trained in PTSD counseling. As I sat and listened to the other spouses the tears began to flow as I began to realize that the anger, irritability and mood swings I saw in my husband were the same emotions that these four ladies described about their husbands.

It was comforting to realize that I was not alone. That the issues I thought were just problems I would have to live with were being faced by many other ladies just like me. It was as if someone turned on the light in the dark room in which I had been confined. Finally, someone understood.

I continued to attend those support group meetings for a short period of time. The doctor put me on medication for depression, and I was doing so well that I thought I did not need the medicine anymore. So I quit taking it.

About a year later, my husband and I had a very heated argument. For the first time, I saw a level of anger in him that I had never seen before. After weeks of replaying the episode in my mind, I realized that I needed someone to help me with the intrusive thoughts for I had begun to sink into that bottomless pit of depression yet again. I reached out to the only person I knew to call which was the therapist I met during the spousal support group two years earlier.

I was deeply depressed again. It seemed that all the years of dealing with PTSD came crashing down around me. This time I could not ignore the signs or the pain that I felt inside.

I had to learn that it was my responsibility to stand up and reclaim my identity in order for me to rise from the depressive state that I found myself. My husband's behavior is not my fault, but the result of some experience in combat that he may not ever share with me. However, it is something he deals with daily ....... and so do I.

While I deal with Secondary PTSD from my marriage, I also deal with PTSD as a result of events that happened to me during my childhood. Therefore, I have the unique opportunity to write this book from both perspectives.

# What is 1 PTSD?

**PTSD** - four letters that changed my life forever even before I knew what the acronym represented.

PTSD is not just the result of combat, but it can result from any traumatic event that happens during a person's life no matter what the age. As with me, the event can occur during childhood but you do not realize that the trauma is the cause of certain emotions and reactions that you have developed until long after you were traumatized. Rape, car accidents, witnessing the death of a loved one, natural disasters are some of the traumatic events that can cause PTSD.

I think that rape is perhaps the most traumatic event that any woman can experience because it is a violation of her body, her spirit, and her will. The trauma intensifies when the woman does not seek a support system to process the trauma but due to the humiliation and embarrassment chooses to try and deal with the situation alone. However, the trauma and its effects will bring on emotions and reactions that the woman does not understand such as anger, low self-esteem, low self-worth, relationship issues, flashbacks, suicidal tendencies, and constant alertness just to name a few.

Everyone is different. The traumatic event that causes PTSD in one individual may not affect another individual in the same way even though they both experienced the same trauma. Also depending on the age of the person and the extent of the trauma, you might completely block the event from your memory for many years only to have it resurface later in life. I experienced one very traumatic event while a child that I completely blocked out of memory. However about 20 years later, the trauma began to slowly resurface in my mind as intrusive thoughts.

Post traumatic stress disorder, better known as PTSD, is a normal reaction to an event that you perceive as life threatening or a horrible experience that leaves you feeling confused, angry or scared. We all have had things happen in our lives that have impacted us in this way. However, we all mentally process things differently. So what may affect one person adversely may not affect another person at all. It is normal for life threatening or life altering events to have a lasting impact on the mental stability of a person. PTSD has been in existence for many years. However, it has been given many different names during its history such as battle fatigue, shell shock, and now PTSD.

Everyone who has PTSD has experienced some type of traumatic event in their lives that has resulted in the fear of losing their life or a feeling of helplessness to stop the horrible event that was occurring to them or around them. These strong emotions have caused changes in the brain that for some individuals will result in PTSD.[1]

The National Center for PTSD[2] lists the following on their website as a means of determining how likely you are to get PTSD as the result of a traumatic event:

- How intense the trauma was or how long it lasted
- If you lost someone you were close to or were hurt
- How close you were to the event
- How strong your reaction was
- How much you felt in control of events
- How much help and support you got after the event

## Symptoms of PTSD

When I was approximately four years old, I was at a neighbor's house when the son came home and got into a heated argument with his dad. Afraid, I ran outside to seek the protection of my mother. The son left only to return later with a stolen rifle and proceeded to shoot at everyone gathered outside. I have basically blocked out all the memories from this event except I still remember my mother and I running through a cornfield. When she would hear the boy shoot the rifle at us, she would tell me to fall to the ground until she was sure the bullets had passed. We never discussed this traumatic event as a family in an attempt to process the trauma.

I never realized the impact that this event had on me until I started counseling sessions. When the therapist asked about events in my past, I recalled this traumatic event in which I felt threatened and scared. I have always been easily startled by noises or even people walking up behind me without my knowledge. For example, I was in a church fellowship hall one Sunday when suddenly a metal folding chair slipped and hit the floor. The sound was extremely loud, and I literally shook so hard that I almost dropped the plate that I was holding in my hand. Never had I associated the incident during my childhood with my reaction to sudden noises or people suddenly appearing from behind me. My husband learned early during our marriage to always announce himself if he came into the house unexpectedly.

The symptoms of PTSD can run the gamut from depression to suicidal tendencies yet not all symptoms are prevalent in everyone. For example, a car tailgating my husband's truck infuriates him where as it does not bother me. I simply keep the same speed or slow down. Just because the person behind me is in a hurry, does not mean that I need to be in a hurry. My husband does not like crowds and neither do I. I prefer to do my shopping when the stores are relatively empty.

Depression is common amongst those suffering from PTSD. Having suffered through two bouts of major depression I know personally that it can be debilitating. There are days when you just want to be left alone. You do not even want to deal with life. Depression can drain you of your energy to the point that getting out of bed seems to be more than you can accomplish. Sleep escapes you and you have low self-esteem. I basically felt that life was not worth the effort and many times I considered suicide. Crying seemed to be the one thing that I could do well.

Depression is a type of pain that is not easily explained. You feel like you are in a black hole, and you can not manage to get out. The pain consumes you, but you fear that no one can understand the torment you are experiencing inside unless they have experienced it also. Therefore a number of depressed people turn to alcohol or other drugs as a coping mechanism. They self-medicate because it is easier than trying to explain to someone the excruciating pain that can come from being in a depressive state.

Isolation is another symptom that seems fairly common especially with combat veterans. It is difficult to talk with someone about the experiences of war that have never been in a war zone. It is not uncommon for veterans to want time alone. When we relocated back to North Carolina, my husband was assigned as the Professor of Military Science at a local college. At the time I was not working professionally, and we had one teenager in high school at home. When my husband came home, I was ready to talk about the day and other events. My husband's desire was to spend time alone after dinner for a couple of hours. I had been alone all day so I had fulfilled my need for isolation but his need for isolation began when he came home. Needless to say this caused some controversy in our relationship. At that time, we did not know that he had PTSD and the many symptoms associated with the disorder.

The one symptom of PTSD that can usually be especially frightening is anger. Some veterans are extremely violent while others are able to suppress their anger somewhat. Suppression of the anger does not lessen its effect when it is expressed. Male veterans when angry may physically abuse the people they love the most – their spouse and children. Breaking chairs, windows or hitting whoever is near is also a common reaction. Some veterans are physically violent while others typically express their anger through emotional and verbal abuse directed at their spouse or children.

It is interesting how some veterans can control their emotional and verbal abuse so that those outside their homes are never suspect of the level of anger that dwells inside the veteran. Individuals outside the home have no idea of the veteran's compressed anger. While dramatic displays of anger are immediately unacceptable and causes the veteran to feel the immediate response to his/her actions, the subtle outbursts of anger displayed in emotional and verbal abuse can do just as must harm to a relationship over time.

Physical abuse seems to draw the greatest outrage because it is immediately evident. However, I classify emotional and verbal abuse as the 'silent killer' that nobody sees, but the impact on the abused person can be very devastating. Short of killing another human being as a result of physical abuse, emotional and verbal abuse can lead to a number of emotional and mental problems for the victim including suicide.

There is no excuse for any type of abuse. If you are in an abusive relationship, I urge you to leave especially if it is a physically abusive relationship because these types of relationships are more prone to result in physical death. If it is an emotionally or verbally abusive relationship, then you can set boundaries of what you will and will not tolerate. If this does not work, then perhaps you should consider if you can mentally deal with the abuse for the remainder of the relationship. While I am not advocating divorce, I believe that divorce is better than death at the hands of the abuser. If you do decide to stay in the relationship, then seek counseling to help you gain the strength and mental stability that you will need to endure the attacks.

Anger is also prevalent in the rape victim. A victim of rape or sexual assault can harbor an intense level of anger not only against her attacker but against men in general. The victim has built an imaginary wall of protection around herself so that she will never be hurt in that manner again. She may seem like an angry person but anger is her defense mechanism. It provides a barrier to keep men, especially, from getting too close. Anger perhaps is the woman's way of controlling the people surrounding her. Generally angry people are avoided rather than embraced. The anger takes the focus off the woman's fear and allows her to temporarily direct the focus of the anger to the targeted person.

I think alienation or avoidance of feelings is the veteran's way of maintaining control of himself and the situation. I can recall the times when the kids and I would surprise my husband with a cover for the truck or a new tool. We had anticipated the excitement and joy he would have. However, we were disappointed when his reaction was more one of being nonchalant. It was disappointing because we were hyped about the surprise. Over the years, I have learned that he just does not get excited about very much. PTSD sufferers have a need to maintain control – control of themselves and their environment. These individuals fear that if they allow themselves to lose control they might not be able to regain control. Therefore they simply avoid showing feelings. To show feelings, would require them to reverse the tactic they have used to numb the memories of war.

As a PTSD sufferer, I know well the anxiety issues that are a constant in our lives. As I mentioned earlier, loud noises greatly disturb me. Lots of veterans are prone to hit the ground or hit the floor prostrate if a loud noise unexpectedly occurs. It is a common reaction to being in a war zone or being attacked.

Sleep is sporadic at best. There are nights when my body is tired but my mind is in mid-day mode. I can not settle my thoughts enough to get sleepy. If I do manage to get to sleep, then it only lasts for a few hours, and I can not get back to sleep. This makes for a very tired and irritable person. The body needs rest but it can not seem to unwind long enough to get the rest it needs. Being in a constant state of alertness denies the body the ability to unwind and sleep appropriately.

Some veterans can not sleep because of constantly checking and rechecking the locks on doors and windows to insure that the family is safe. My husband would go throughout the house at night checking and rechecking door locks. We have motion detector lights outside our home. This makes me feel safer because no one can come to my front door at night without my knowing that someone or something is outside and within a certain distance of my front door.

For many, sleep is an unpleasant experience. It allows intrusive thoughts to enter the mind through dreams. The veteran make wake up and not realize for a moment that he or she is not in the combat zone. The rape victim might wake up screaming thinking she is being attacked again. The car accident victim may wake up thinking he is back in the car accident again.

Panic/anxiety attacks are a common reaction to the stress placed on the body during an episode of intrusive thoughts re-entering the mind. Intrusive thoughts are simply replaying in your mind the traumatic event. I experienced a panic attack while in my therapist's office. I had just had a session that morning where I told him about the events that had occurred to me during my childhood. Remembering was more than I could mentally deal with.

After entertaining suicidal thoughts, my therapist had me return to his office. I had only been in his office a few minutes when I felt the attack start. Fortunately, I was with him. He later told me it was a panic attack. It was one of the worst experiences of my life. I had actually been hospitalized for a panic attack three years earlier. I know, from experience, how intrusive thoughts can affect a person. I know the need to keep anxiety under control.

As I mentioned earlier, intrusive thoughts are simply replaying the traumatic event in your mind over and over again. It is as if someone keeps pushing the replay button, and you have no control. I can see my Mom and me running through the cornfield and hitting the ground when the gun was fired. I can see the image of me lying on the floor being raped when I was eight or nine years old. My mind has blocked out the person's face who raped me. However, I can see myself lying there, and I remember the intense pain that I felt. These are some of my intrusive thoughts. Short glimpses of pain suffered at the hands of two different attackers.

There are many symptoms of PTSD. While I have my own symptoms that I deal with daily from PTSD, veterans and other PTSD sufferers deal with their own specific set of symptoms. For example, some veterans are physically abusive and others are not. Your symptoms depend to some degree on the traumatic event that you experienced, and how quickly you sought help after the traumatic event to help you process what you had witnessed.

There is no cure for PTSD. It is a disorder that many people must deal with daily for the rest of their lives. The symptoms might improve. However, the disorder is incurable. The individual diagnosed with PTSD can learn coping skills through counseling. However, you never know when or what will trigger the next episode, but hopefully when it happens, you will have developed the skills to cope.

With the increased knowledge of PTSD, more therapists and counselors are professionally trained to deal with the disorder. If you or someone you love displays any of the symptoms of PTSD, I encourage you to contact the nearest Veterans Administration Center or seek out a therapist or counselor who is trained in PTSD counseling. Your life and the lives of others may depend on it.

# What is Secondary PTSD?

Individuals that care for trauma patients can and do often experience symptoms very similar to the symptoms of the trauma patient. This is a concern with all caregivers especially in professions such as counselors, therapists, firemen, or first response police officers who respond to crime scenes involving the death or suicide of children or teenagers. My son has been asthmatic since age two. However, I still feel fear, anxiety and lack of control whenever he experiences an asthma attack. Just as my son feels a lack of control to be able to breathe, I feel a lack of control in being able to help him during the attack.

Secondary PTSD as discussed in this book will focus on the caring of a veteran who suffers from PTSD. This disorder is generally associated with the spouse or the caregiver of the veteran. Basically, Secondary PTSD is very similar to PTSD. The main difference is the caregiver's symptoms are secondary because she did not experience the trauma directly but rather indirectly from what the veteran has chosen to verbally communicate to her regarding his traumatic event.

A Veteran may choose not to talk about the traumas of war to his spouse because he thinks the spouse would never understand because she was not actually in the war zone. I think this perhaps is true of most traumatic events. While you can try to explain the trauma that you experienced, another person can not truly understand the emotional aspect of what you endured unless they themselves have been through the same or a very similar situation.

PTSD is not a contagious disease. However, overtime as the caregiver of a veteran you begin to unknowingly assume some of the same symptoms as the veteran. Your view of life is gradually altered by the issues of trauma that your veteran is dealing with daily. As the spouse, you are dealing with the trauma issues daily because you have automatically slipped into the role as his caregiver by virtue of being his spouse.

Spouses who suffer Secondary PTSD often describe it as "walking on eggshells". You are always trying to stay one step ahead of your husband by attempting to eliminate those things that could possibly cause him to become upset. When he does become upset, you are trying to find ways to fix the problem. Thus you live in a state of high alert. Always anticipating what might happen and trying to find ways to prevent what is often the inevitable. We become a lot like the soldier in combat – always anticipating the attack of the enemy. Despite your every attempt to make life perfect, you are still quite often berated and yelled at by the person that you are constantly trying to help.

Therefore you end up feeling hurt, angry, and alone. The one problem I faced was I had no one to talk to when this happened, and I feel that a lot of spouses dealing with these issues can relate to the feeling of "I am the only one". I was not able to effectively handle the emotional side of failing to meet my husband's needs or being able to understand his mood swings.

I took his mood swings personal as if it was the result of something I had done or failed to do. My self-worth and self-esteem hit rock bottom and depression was the end result.

It became emotionally exhausting trying to figure out the right thing to do when everything I did seemed to be wrong. I became unhappy and quite frankly just did not want to continue living if this was what the remainder of my life was going to be like. I felt isolated, helpless, and angry – some of the same issues that those who suffer PTSD deal with on a daily basis.

Communicating my feelings to my husband was not an option. I just endured his mood swings and never let him see me cry or tell him how much I hurt inside. After years of living this way, I now know that I should have been more forthcoming with him rather than trying to protect him by keeping everything inside. Emotionally and mentally I reached my limit, and the end result was a constant desire to find peace. The only way I could envision this peace was to end my life.

While it is becoming more common to diagnose the spouse as having Secondary PTSD, I believe that many spouses of PTSD veterans also suffer from PTSD as well. Spouses that are abused whether physically, emotionally, or verbally are experiencing direct trauma. This is not trauma that they have heard about. This is one or more traumatic events that have happened to them directly. The abuse is the result of the traumatic event the PTSD veteran suffered, but it is a direct trauma to the spouse. She is now the victim of her own traumatic event.

Now the spouse is in the caregiver role of the person that has abused her. She now faces many of the same symptoms that her veteran spouse has from his traumatic event coupled with the issues that have surfaced as the result of being an unappreciated caregiver. This is a role that she did not ask for but was thrust into simply because she thought that somehow she could make things better for her veteran husband.

## Seeking Help for Secondary PTSD

Unfortunately, there are few resources available to assist the spouse of a veteran suffering from PTSD. The military is offering classes to those active duty soldiers and their spouses who have been in a combat zone. However, the veteran spouse has to pursue information and treatment on her own.

The Veterans Administration (VA) system is currently not organized to handle the veteran spouse unless the veteran himself is enrolled in the VA system and is actively pursuing treatment. This presents a problem since many veterans think they do not have a problem and the issues in their spouse and the family is the fault of everyone but the veteran.

If only you were a better wife or mother. If only the children did not make so much noise. If only you kept the house cleaner. If only you had dinner prepared when I got home. The 'if only' list goes on and on. The veteran perceives that everybody has a problem but himself. Therefore, he refuses to enroll in the VA programs and the spouse is denied any services in the VA system and must seek professional help elsewhere.

The primary problem with seeking professional counseling elsewhere is finding a counselor or therapist that is trained in PTSD and Secondary PTSD and understands the idiosyncrasies of military life. If the family is already experiencing financial difficulties, then this will probably prevent the spouse from seeking the help she needs. Also the veteran himself may prohibit the spouse from seeking help.

Emotional support is very important when dealing with Secondary PTSD. As I mentioned earlier, I felt isolated and therefore felt that no one could understand the stress that I was under. As a caregiver I had basically allowed his life to become my life. I did not have friends and basically had no idea of who I was anymore.

It is imperative that you develop friendships and if possible, join a support group. If there is not a group in your area, you might want to start one if there are a number of veteran spouses in your area. Even if there is only one, then you have someone who understands what you are going through. You should not feel guilty about enjoying time with friends. This will give you the opportunity to think about things other than your personal situation and allow you to connect with other people.

Over indulging in alcohol and/or drugs is not the answer when coping with this disorder. It only creates more problems for you and the family. Even if your veteran spouse uses alcohol and/or drugs, do not join him in this worthless coping mechanism.

It is important that you take care of yourself. Take time to do some things that you enjoy such as reading, gardening, crafts, or taking long walks. I enjoy going to the bookstore or to the coffee shop and reading with a cup of coffee. It is a simple outing that costs little but refreshes my mind and gets me out of my home environment for a period of time.

# The Effect of PTSD on Relationships

The family is gathering at your Mother's home for the annual Christmas dinner. You have discussed it with your PTSD Veteran husband, and he agreed to go. So, just as you are about to call the kids to leave, your husband announces that he is not going.

So you have two choices: 1) Stay home to accommodate his desire not to go, or 2) Go to the family dinner and leave him home alone.

Some spouses will choose to stay home, calling Mom at the last minute with some fake excuse as to why the family can not attend. Other spouses will choose to leave their husband at home alone and attend the event offering some lame excuse as to why the husband chose to stay home. It does not matter which choice you choose it makes for an angry spouse who has to make a choice to stay home with a husband who may isolate himself while you are there or to once again deal with a husband and his broken promise to be part of a family event. The one issue not mentioned is what do you tell the children in either situation?

Many individuals that suffer from PTSD will avoid crowds at all cost. The mall is off limits. Family gatherings are off limits. Even living too close to neighbors is off limits. PTSD sufferers need space and quite often just want to be left alone. There are some Veterans who become loners and are constantly moving. Other Veterans choose to relocate to a remote place with lots of unoccupied land. Some Veterans can not stay employed for very long while others choose jobs at night which eliminates interacting with family and aids in avoiding nightly social gatherings.

My husband does not like crowds and neither do I. This is one symptom of PTSD that we both possess. For me, crowds create anxiety, a need to break free, to find a place that is less stressful with less people. It seems I lose an element of control. I do not like people invading my personal space. Therefore, I prefer to shop when others are either at home or at work.

Anger is a major concern for the Veteran. Many times when we were having family dinners in our home, my husband would become irritable and angry a couple of hours before the guest were to arrive. Initially, I did not understand the mood swing until I began to understand PTSD.

Family gatherings in our home invaded his space. He felt a loss of control. He is not one to sit and talk after dinner. Normally, he excuses himself from the dinner table and finds comfort in front of the television where he becomes completely engrossed in a television program thereby eliminating the requirement to talk. So while the rest of the family is still around the dinner table talking long after the meal is over, my husband has isolated himself to the family room where he normally has the television so loud that we struggle to talk in the adjoining room.

Not wanting to upset my husband while family is over, I generally do not say anything about how loud he has the television because I do not want to deal with his backlash or have the family witness an angry outburst. I have learned to pick and choose my battles.

From personal experience, depression has quite often been the reason I absolutely hated gatherings of any kind whether with family or friends. I was involved in activities at church that I removed myself from. Many Sundays I did not even want to go to church because I knew people would be there, and I simply just did not feel like dealing with people. It was emotionally and mentally taxing and difficult for me to smile when inside I felt a constant need to escape. My instinct was to get out of there as quickly as possible. I just wanted to be alone.

My family, my one close friend, and the people at church knew I was different somehow. One lady told me that I had lost my sparkle. I could not tell them that I was clinically depressed and that I suffered from PTSD and secondary PTSD and that it took every ounce of energy I could muster just to go out in public.

I, like so many Veterans, have faced situations that nobody can understand unless they too have experienced the trauma of war or rape. It becomes easier to just not associate with people. This eliminates the requirement to offer an explanation to people when they realize that the smile you are wearing is simply a mask that can not hide the sadness they see in your eyes. My desire was to be alone. This prevented the need to pretend.

I isolated myself from my family and church members. I never really had friends so that was not an issue. At the time, I was working outside the home, but my job was such that I spent the majority of my time alone at my desk – which was perfect for me. I did not have to talk to anybody.

Unfortunately, I reduced communication with my adult children. I never knew they had noticed until my son mentioned that he realized that I did not call or text him as often as I once did. I distanced myself from my mom who called my husband to see if I was angry with her and if that was the reason I had quit calling her. My husband and I could ride in the same vehicle for an hour without speaking. I simply had nothing to say. It was not that there was nothing on my mind because my mind was full of thoughts. Intrusive thoughts that repeated themselves over and over again, but I chose to stay in my own silent world.

Families quite often do not understand PTSD. In my case, neither my family nor my husband's family is aware that we both have PTSD. We simply have not told them. Only our son is aware, but no one else.

Even though we have chosen to not share this information with our families, I think it would have been beneficial if we did. It would have alleviated the need to pretend on my part that everything was normal when I was contemplating suicide moments before talking with one of them on the phone. It would have explained the empty stares and lack of enjoyment when we were together as a family. It would have helped my family to understand why I isolated myself and just wanted to be left alone. I did not want to talk to anybody because quite frankly I had nothing to say.

I find it is often hard to truly open up to someone. Quite often I feel the need to keep my thoughts to myself. Therefore I have never had a close friend until recently. Even my son asked me recently why I never had friends when he was growing up. This is a common attribute of many individuals who survive traumatic events. It becomes easier to not get too close to someone. The fear of getting too close and truly opening up to someone removes some of the control that the individual has over his emotions. It became easier to isolate myself and not get to close to anyone. (Quite often this can even be an issue between husbands and wives as well.) For me it was easier to isolate myself with my intrusive thoughts and emotional numbing which resulted in anxiety, anger and depression. It is a vicious cycle that when left untreated just keeps repeating its self.

## Support for the PTSD Survivor and Those They Love

One of the greatest things a PTSD survivor can do is first seek counseling for himself or herself. I sought counseling when I realized that I could not deal with my issues alone. The road of depression was not new to me. I am forever indebted to my initial therapist who quite often I could subconsciously feel him holding me back from stepping off the cliff of suicide.

Counseling allowed me, as it will other PTSD sufferers, to better understand the symptoms of this illness and learn how to cope with situations when they arise. I truly believe that anyone who suffers from PTSD should seek counseling. It is not an illness that you can ignore, and why live a defeated life especially when there are individuals trained specifically to help you deal with your individual problems.

While it is imperative that the trauma survivor seek counseling, it is also important for the immediate family to seek counseling as well. This can include the spouse and children and also any adult children caring for an older parent with PTSD.

There is an abundance of information available about PTSD and its effects on trauma survivors. I highly recommend that families and friends take the time to research the illness in order to gain a better understanding of PTSD and its many symptoms. I have included a listing of websites at the back of this book that offers valuable information on PTSD.

It was not until I began to do my own research on PTSD that I began to understand my husband's behavior. Instead of just assuming that I had no control over my life, I began to research PTSD and find ways to help me better deal with my husband's symptoms. I can not control him, but I can control how I respond to him. While there is an abundance of information readily available for the Veteran, there is limited information for the spouse available. Therefore, hopefully, this book will provide some insight to the world of PTSD that you now find yourself residing.

As a person who has suffered clinical depression from PTSD and secondary PTSD, I wanted someone that I could trust and openly express my thoughts and feelings. Someone that I could talk to about what I had experienced. Someone who would truly listen and not judge me. Someone that I felt cared about me. Someone that I could trust. My therapists and my psychiatrist have become those special people that allowed me to share my innermost thoughts in one on one sessions. While individual sessions worked better for me, support group sessions might work better for others.

All PTSD sufferers need someone. Quite often Veterans find support in groups at the VA Clinic that allows them to talk through their issues and provide support to each other. Family members, caregivers, and especially spouses quite often lack this support system. Therefore, we have to be proactive in educating ourselves on PTSD and finding support groups that can understand the struggles that families and friends of trauma survivors must deal with.

Living with PTSD and secondary PTSD is extremely difficult. The absolute best thing I ever did for myself was to seek counseling. Life is still a daily struggle, but with medications and coping skills I am better able to handle my symptoms.

I urge you if you have a loved one or a friend whom you suspect has PTSD to encourage him or her to seek evaluation by a medical professional that can get them into the proper treatment programs according to their needs.

I urge you as the family member or friend to seek counseling for yourself if you are the caregiver or at least become knowledgeable of PTSD.

# The Effect of PTSD on the Spouse

*Why does life have to hurt so bad? I am tired of the pain that is deep inside that I think I have learned to cope with only to have it mutate and return again.*

*The people I hold dear don't truly understand how I feel. They can't. No one knows what I feel inside but me.*

*The loneliness, the despair, the lack of accomplishment, the low self-esteem. If you have been successful there is no way you can understand my pain of rejection. Knowing that I am capable but no one will give me a chance. One look at my resume says it all.*

*For 20 plus years, I devoted myself to my husband and my kids. Now I feel like I have nothing. Nothing but a persistent pain that keeps me from moving forward. But I don't have anything to move forward to.*

*Somewhere I lost myself, my dreams, my desires. Somewhere I lost me, and I don't know how to relate to this person that I have become.*

*One minute I am fine and the next minute I am a bucket of tears. The seemingly happy moments are only a masquerade to cover the pain.*

*I keep treading water trying to stay afloat. But I am slowly sinking. Not able to decide what is best for me. Not wanting to make the wrong decision. I am indecisive. Wish I could live both lives to see which one I like better. Unfortunately, life doesn't work that way. You live with the choices you make. Good or bad.*

*I am someone who can be lonely in a crowded room. I sit quietly listening, thinking, but never contributing to the conversation. After all what I have to say probably isn't important or eventually someone else will say what I was thinking.*

*So why bother. Just stay in my own world. Nobody notices anyway.*

*What is peace? Is peace ever possible? I only wish I knew. I thought of suicide, but I don't want to leave that scar on my children's heart for the remainder of their lives. I can't even die in peace.*

*Just please take the pain away. Let me find peace.*

Does peace exist for the Veteran spouse? I live in a world of mood swings, isolation, numbing, depression, suicidal thoughts and the list goes on. However, since I suffer from PTSD and Secondary PTSD, I am constantly bombarded either with my own PTSD symptoms or Secondary PTSD symptoms. The challenge is dealing not only with my own issues but those of a PTSD spouse as well. If I knew what day of the week a symptom would surface in my husband, I would be better prepared to cope. However, the symptoms surface when I least expect them and many times a single word or statement is all it takes for my husband to migrate into one of the many symptoms of PTSD. This in turn leaves me feeling guilty that something I said or done has caused him to seek shelter inside himself.

This does not sound like a peaceful way to live. I am constantly mindful of my words, my actions, everything. This is comparable to walking around in a minefield and you never know if your next step will be the one where everything explodes. I live in a state of constant alertness.

Last Sunday, I wore a new dress to church and one of the ladies told me that I looked stunning. While having dinner with my husband the next evening, I mentioned the comment, and I added that this lady is my number one fan. My husband immediately changed from being talkative to being non-talkative and isolated himself for the remainder of the evening.

An innocent statement, so I thought; but for him it was a trigger. Why? I do not know. Once again in my efforts to successfully navigate the minefield, I had inadvertently stepped on a mine.

I kept repeating in my mind that his behavior was not my fault, but I have not reached the point of actually believing what I keep telling myself. It is a continuous battle, but it is one that I must win if I am to survive mentally.

My focus has always been my husband and my children. Their needs became my needs. I became the caregiver, the peacemaker, and in many cases the glue that held everything together so that people on the outside of the four walls we call home thought we were just a normal family with the normal issues that any family faces.

But what happens to you, when the glue starts to dry and crack? At some point, you just can not be everything to everybody anymore. So what happens to you?

For me, I crumbled. The depression that I had tried to keep at bay finally hit me like a boulder. The years of verbal and emotional abuse by my husband had finally taken its toll. I started the downward slide into the black hole that I call the abyss. It seemed that my fall was gaining speed and the walls of the black pit I now found myself were slippery and provided nothing to hold onto. Not only was my downward spiral from the secondary PTSD but also from the childhood PTSD that I had never dealt with before.

In my effort as a spouse to take care of everybody else, I neglected myself. My primary focus was taking care of everyone else at the detriment of ignoring my needs. I had learned to turn inside the hurt and humiliation from the abuse of my husband not allowing him to see the pain I was feeling. I learned to cry inside while smiling on the outside. There was no one to help me. I gradually reached the end of my rope; I reached my breaking point. I no longer was the glue that held everything together.

I then began to question myself and wondered if life as it had been was worth the effort. Why do I have to constantly walk on eggshells to avoid the next explosion or period of isolation? Who was caring for my needs? There was no one to care for me. My needs were not being met. I had become someone controlled by the actions of my spouse. I did whatever it took to avoid my husband falling prey to the symptoms of PTSD.

I woke up one morning to reality after many counseling sessions and asked myself if my love for my husband was enough to make me want to live like this the rest of my life or for my own mental stability should I walk away. A wise therapist once said that sometimes love is not enough. Your Veteran husband may truly love you, but if he abuses you in anyway then his love may actually result in death if you choose to stay in an abusive relationship.

For many Veteran spouses, this becomes a question that you will mentally and emotionally toss back and forth sometimes for years. Quite often never knowing what is best for you, or knowing what is best but never having the courage to walk out the door. Before counseling, I could never imagine life alone. My self-esteem and self-worth had been devalued by the abuse to the point that I felt I could not survive without my husband no matter the extent of the abuse I suffered. It took counseling for me to believe in my self again – for me to believe that I actually am capable of standing alone if I have to.

Your husband does not have PTSD by choice, but it was the result of some traumatic event. An event that occurred as a result of him doing the job he had been ordered to do. He did not have a choice.

So you feel sympathy for him; because his having PTSD is not his fault. Therefore you feel that you should stay because leaving would seem inappropriate. Unloving. You would be leaving your husband for a reason that really was not his fault. However, the question remains can you continue to live in an environment of uncertainty. Where do you draw the line to determine what you will endure for love and what becomes too much to bear?

Many spouses can not decide to stay or go. They cling to the hope that some how their husband will change; he will get better. It is possible that the Veteran can learn coping skills through counseling, but PTSD is incurable. It is a lifelong illness. However, many Veterans believe that the problem does not lie with them, but it is everybody else that has problems and issues that they need to deal with.

My childhood traumas still affect me today. Intrusive thoughts, loud noises, and people approaching me from behind still cause a certain degree of anxiety for me.

However, I have learned to manage my reaction so that I can deal with the situations in a more realistic manner.

While I have learned mechanisms through counseling to help me cope with the symptoms, the traumatic events are forever branded in my mind. It has become a part of who I am. It was not a choice that I made, but rather a choice that someone else made to harm me. Unfortunately, I have to live with the choice that each person who attacked me made. It is not fair that I am forever dealing with an illness that controls who I am. I had no choice in the matter. The attackers made a choice that I am forced to live with everyday.

Does the spouse of a PTSD Veteran ever find peace? Unfortunately, I do not think it is possible to have total peace in this life whether you are married to a Veteran or not. Walking around in a minefield for the rest of your life certainly does not provide an image of peace, but of constant uncertainty and pain.

However, being married to a spouse with PTSD introduces challenges and struggles that the wife of a non-PTSD spouse does not have to face or deal with. This is why it is so important to become part of a group of other spouses that can understand your specific struggles. For example, why is my husband always angry? Why does he prefer to be alone than to spend time with me his wife? Why does everything I do seem to be wrong?

There are many spouses going through the same issues as you. It was only in a support group of other Veteran spouses that I learned that my life was different because of PTSD. My husband's many behavioral tendencies were not my fault, but a byproduct of PTSD.

If you choose to stay with your Veteran spouse, you will eventually develop coping techniques that will give you moments of peace. It is those moments that will help you through the emotional roller coaster that is lurking just around the corner.

As for me, I decided that I will not live the rest of my life like I have lived the past. My mental stability is more important to me. I would be of no use to my children mentally incapacitated, and I do not want to hurt them by committing suicide. So things must change. My depressive state has been a living hell, but I have emerged stronger from the experience through counseling.

# The Effect of PTSD on the Children

What about the children? Does PTSD only affect the Veteran and the spouse? Absolutely not. PTSD can and usually does affect every person living in the home to some degree. No one is exempt. The children may not be affected the same way as the spouse, but they are affected none the less.

The main concern with children is they quite often do not understand why Dad acts as he does. They do not understand why Dad is always angry or criticizes them all the time or why their parents seem to argue a lot. It is even more difficult for a child living in a home where the Veteran over indulges in alcohol or physically abuses the spouse and sometimes the children as well. Children may have problems verbalizing their frustrations and anger. So children of Veterans with PTSD may resort to acting out their frustrations through inappropriate behaviors.

How does a mother explain to her children that Dad acts the way he does because he has PTSD when the mother barely understands PTSD herself. This is the very reason that I initiated my own research to better understand PTSD so that I could help my children understand their Dad's behavior better. There simply has not been enough research done to understand the effects of PTSD on children and how it can affect them later in life. However, whether or not the research exists, I know that PTSD does affect the children living in a home with a father who suffers from PTSD.

Quite often I think adults are misguided in their view of children's ability to perceive when something is not right. Just because they are children does not mean they are not aware of their surroundings. Too many times an adult's life is shaped by the events that happened to him or her when he or she was a child. I personally can identify with the fact that events that occurred before I reached the age of ten have had a great impact on me as an adult.

Therefore children might not ever ask why Dad does not want to be around them or why they can not have friends over when Dad is home. The questions may never be verbalized, but you can be sure that the questions do exist in the mind of the child.

When my kids were growing up, I tried to keep the number of kids in my home to a minimum especially if it was close to the time my husband came home from work. Whenever I found out he was going on a temporary duty (TDY) assignment, I would tell the kids they could invite a friend over to spend the night while their Dad was out of town.

How do you explain the Veteran's behavior when your daughter asks, "Why won't Daddy come to any of my games?" or the son does not understand why his Dad will not go outside and play catch with him?

I can remember many Friday nights rushing home from work, cooking dinner, and then rushing to my daughter's games to support her. My son did not want to go to the games so he was left home to wash the dishes and wait for his Dad to come home. Many nights I would return home only to find my son and my husband watching the same television program. However, my son would have spent the evening in the family room alone while my husband was in the bedroom with the door closed preparing for class and watching television. I am sure this type situation has unfolded in many homes numerous times.

It is ironic when the Veteran blames the wife for not allowing him to be part of the family when the kids were growing up. In reality, the wife would have welcomed a more involved husband and father. It was the Veteran that pulled away, but he blames his wife when the children go to her to meet their needs instead of their father. Again a common symptom of PTSD is to place the blame on someone else.

When my husband's PTSD impacted one of our children, I generally became the peacemaker talking to the child trying to help them understand why their Dad acted as he did and trying to make their pain go away. I would also talk with my husband trying to get him to give the child some slack. The problem was at this point I truly did not understand why my husband acted as he did because he had not yet been diagnosed with PTSD which made life for me even harder.

Children are more perceptive than we think. In retrospect, I am sure my children knew that I was hurting just like them. It seems that I was caught between my husband and my children. I became the buffer that was being pushed from both sides. However, as a Mom, it impacts my very being to see my child hurting. So I did what I thought was best at the time. If I had known about PTSD, I would have handled things differently. I did the best that I could with the limited knowledge that I had.

*Erica David*

## Explaining PTSD to Children

It is imperative that children are educated about PTSD. You can not assume that the child does not notice that something is amiss especially when their friends are not experiencing the same reactions from their non-PTSD dad. Even toddlers are aware when situations change or people change. Talking with children about PTSD better enables them to know how to handle their Dad's actions and reactions and not to just assume that their Dad's response is their fault.

Educating yourself first as the spouse and then educating your children is essential to learning to live with a PTSD Veteran. If the Veteran is willing, he can have a discussion with the children to educate them on PTSD according to the following points as taken from the National Center for PTSD website[3]:

1.  Be honest and listen to what they have to say
2.  Tell them it is okay to ask questions. Ask them how they're feeling, and let them know that their concerns are important.
3.  Make sure they feel safe, secure, and loved. They may be afraid that something bad is going to happen.
4.  Provide information about PTSD. Let them know what it is, how you got it, and how you can recover.
5.  Encourage a good support system of friends outside your family. Get them involved in school activities or youth programs in the community.
6.  Don't promise that your PTSD is going to go away soon. Instead, talk about how treatment

can help you feel better. It's okay if you don't
have all the answers.

7. Be as positive as you can. Your kids will notice
how you react in difficult situations, which can
influence their reactions.

If the Veteran does not want to or will not have the
conversation with the children, then I implore you as the
spouse to follow the seven steps above to discuss PTSD with
your children.

## How to Explain PTSD According to a Child's Age

Obviously, you can not explain PTSD to a toddler the
same way you would to a teenager. You must determine
what your child is capable of comprehending at his or her
age. However, keep in mind that children quite often have
the ability to comprehend much more than we as adults
think they can understand.

The following age guidelines are taken from the article
'Helping Children Understand PTSD[4]:

1. Infants and toddlers
   This age group notices that they are not receiving
   the love that they once received from the PTSD
   parent. This group, while aware of the change in
   the level of love received, is confused and much
   too young to understand PTSD. It is important to
   protect the child's feelings as they may not want to
   spend time with their Dad who has withdrawn his
   love from them to some degree.

2. Preschoolers and Kindergarteners
   This is definitely the age of questions. Often answers
   are followed by a continuous "why", which can drive
   even a sane person to become a little emotionally
   distraught. This age group like the preceding age

group can not grasp the meaning of PTSD, but they may resort to calling the PTSD Dad either good or evil depending on the situation. This age group does not know when the PTSD Veteran has reached his limit and all questions need to cease. Just one more "why" could be the one thing that causes an angry outburst or worse from the PTSD Veteran.

Children at this age can be taught that when Daddy is having a bad day to just play quietly in their room and do not ask questions. It is also important to talk with the child after an outburst to explain that it was not the child's fault.

3. School-Age Children

In today's society, children of this age group have probably either read about PTSD or heard about it from the media. While this group may be somewhat familiar with the term PTSD, it is still important that you as the mother talk individually with your children to answer any questions that they may have and to try to alleviate any fears they may have as well.

Encourage the child to research PTSD or the two of you can research it together. Also encourage your child to pursue interests outside the home such as sports, academic clubs, music lessons, friends, and trustworthy adults the child can talk to for advice. Quite often a child facing a seemingly insurmountable obstacle will open up to an adult who is not a parent much quicker because the child feels more comfortable talking with someone other that his or her parent.

Do not allow a PTSD Veteran to be an escape goat for not punishing your child when he has violated a family rule. It is easy to fall into that trap that the child suffers so much emotionally at home with a PTSD Dad that you do not want to punish the child when he or she has obviously done something wrong. One way to handle this is to let the child help decide the punishment. The child will usually decide on a punishment much harsher that you would have given.

Another important point for this age group is to have the child and the PTSD Dad spend time together on the days when the Veteran is doing well. This will help to keep the Veteran active in the child's life and help to deepen the bond of father and child.

4.  Teenagers
    The teenage years are difficult enough without having the added pressure of a Dad with PTSD.

I have two adult children that survived the teenage years with a PTSD Dad. It was not easy. Mainly because their Dad was not diagnosed with PTSD until my daughter was in college and my son was a freshman in high school. So I was not able to talk with them about PTSD earlier in their growing years because I had just heard the term, and I actually had no idea what it meant. It was only after much research that I began to better understand how PTSD had affected my family.

Teenagers definitely know what is going on and may become angry at the Dad for how he treats their Mother. The teenager may choose to avoid his Dad or have little interactions with him. I can recall many nights when I sat in the family room while my two children and my husband were each in their separate bedrooms.

The problematic issue occurs when the teenagers go to Mom to meet their needs and bypass Dad because they are avoiding the potential angry outburst or the criticism from their Dad. While the teenager is protecting herself, it causes the Dad to become angry with the Mother ultimately accusing her of not allowing him to be a part of the family or not allowing him to fulfill the role of Dad.

I would talk with my son when I learned of PTSD and try to help him better understand his Dad's behavior. My daughter was away at college, and I never discussed the subject with her. Since I was one of those Mothers that the children usually came to when they needed something, I began to encourage my son to go to his Dad. I tried to step back and allow them to form a father and son relationship. I must admit, it was not always easy, but my son usually would internalize his Dad's angry outbursts and criticism. My son generally did not respond.

My concern is the effect that PTSD has had on both my children. It was not their fault or my fault or their Dad's fault. None of us knew about PTSD. All I knew is that after he spent over four months in the desert during the Gulf War, the man that returned home was different from my husband that left two days after Christmas four months earlier.

Many military kids today are growing up in homes affected by PTSD. The child becomes accustomed to many angry outbursts, sometimes abuse and other issues resulting from having a PTSD Veteran as a Dad or Mother. In many cases the child sees himself as the reason for the parent's anger, or a teenager may be angry with Dad for how he treats the Mother and sometimes angry with the Mother for not standing up for herself and for the kids. Children may be too young to understand PTSD, but children understand anger at a very young age.

Low self-esteem, low self-worth, depression, violent outbursts are just a few of the issues that can affect a child growing up with a parent that suffers from PTSD. Some children suffer physical abuse at the hands of a PTSD parent. The child may not know how or choose to not verbalize his thoughts which results in the child internalizing his thoughts only to have them resurface later in life.

Less research has been done on children growing up with a PTSD parent than on spouses of PTSD Veterans. There has been a tremendous effort by the military to understand and provide for the Veteran with PTSD. However, not enough effort has gone into understanding the effect of PTSD on the children. Active duty families attend some classes to inform them about PTSD and its effects, but the retired military family is left to handle the issues on their own with little to no support from the very organization that should provide as much assistance as possible considering how the Veteran was exposed to events that resulted in PTSD.

Since PTSD has the potential to be devastating not only to the Veteran but to his family as well, it would seem plausible that this knowledge would have been more than adequate for the military to better educate not only the Veteran but the family as well.

# Establishing Boundaries

If we tolerate abuse, we get abused. If we tolerate anger, we are treated in an angry manner. If we tolerate a controlling individual, then we will be controlled. If we say 'yes', when we really mean 'no', then we tolerate the pain of our own weakness to set a boundary of what we will and will not tolerate.

A spouse with PTSD may use his illness as justification for his actions. I have heard remarks such as 'I will always have mood swings', 'if you had not kept talking I would not have had to hit you'. Notice that the problem always lies with someone else or something else. The PTSD Veteran often thinks he has no issues, does not need counseling, and can not understand what your problem is with him. Bottom line, your biggest problem is not your spouse per se, but the symptoms associated with PTSD that often invade your relationship along with a PTSD spouse that refuses to admit that his illness is causing any problems. It does not cause problems as long as the Veteran's wife is willing to tolerate the abusive behavior of the PTSD spouse. It is when the wife begins to set boundaries that all hell breaks loose because the Veteran starts losing control.

When I first thought about this chapter on boundaries, I thought it would focus more on setting boundaries for my husband. However, as I began to research this topic, I began to understand that the boundaries were not to be set for my husband, but they were to be boundaries that I set for myself. I can not control him, but I can control what I am willing to tolerate and what I will not tolerate. Therefore setting personal boundaries is my way of protecting me. I have to protect my heart, my mind, and my will because others will only seek to take from me and abuse me if I allow them.

Setting boundaries has been very difficult for me. I still want to eliminate the boundary when I have to deal with the anger or resentment that results from establishing a boundary. However, I have to realize that my husband's anger is his problem and not mine. I am learning to not make other people's problems my problems.

## What are Boundaries?

There are many ways to think of boundaries. I think of the commercials where the roommates establish boundaries by drawing a line on the floor down the middle of the room. The boundary of your property is another example. You control what happens on your property but you can not intrude on your neighbor's property and start planting flowers or erecting fences.

Another example is the boundary you establish when you park your car. You lock the doors establishing a boundary. If someone chooses to enter your vehicle through illegal means, then that person has violated your boundary and must suffer the consequences.

One of my boundaries, which invisible to others, is what I refer to as my personal space. People sometimes think I need them to get within inches of my face for me to understand or hear what they are saying. My tendency is to back up because that person has just invaded my invisible but very real boundary that I have established for myself. I think many people have a personal space boundary that they do not like invaded.

Boundaries help us to know what belongs to us so that we can protect what is ours.

## What about Boundaries in Relationships?

In order for relationships to thrive, boundaries must be established. If boundaries are not established, then the initial attraction that the couple had is not enough to sustain a long lasting relationship. The couple never will truly know each other and never learn how to grow as a couple. For a happy, successful marriage to survive, it must have established boundaries otherwise one or both spouses will ultimately resort to tolerating things that he or she wishes would change but the spouse feels helpless in bringing about change – simply because she believes that marriage is about tolerating the abuse, anger, drunkenness or controlling nature of a spouse. After all, it has not been that long ago when abused women were told by well meaning mothers and sisters to go back to their abusive husbands because it is just something that happens in some marriages. Hopefully, today that lie is not being told to any woman. A man simply because he is your husband does not have the right to hit you or threaten you. It is a crime.

Marriage was never meant to be a relationship where one person defines the marriage and the spouse simply must submit. Marriage is a relationship where two people should love each other enough to respect each other as equals.

Marriage is not a place where one spouse should live in fear of what the other spouse might do if he becomes angry. In my opinion, this is not a loving relationship but has become a controlled environment where love no longer exists.

I mentioned earlier about my invisible boundary which I referred to as my personal space. We can easily understand those boundaries that we can see or touch, but what about the boundaries we can not touch or see.

One boundary area that has been particularly difficult for me is my use of words. Due to events that occurred during childhood, I never really allowed other people to get to know me. I would say what I thought they wanted to hear. To me, my opinion did not matter. I can remember many times my husband would ask my opinion and my response was usually what I thought he wanted me to say not how I actually felt about the situation.

This lack of boundary resulted in my not observing the boundary of truth. In failing to tell my husband how I actually felt, I misled him. Since he can not read my mind, he thought I was happy and content with whatever the situation happened to be. In reality, the smile on the outside was a cover for the pain or disappointment I felt inside.

Sometimes the boundary of distance is needed. After suffering major depression, I needed emotional distance to heal. My husband moved into another bedroom to give me space and time alone. My therapist was not very supportive of me moving out of the house on my own because I was extremely suicidal at the time. So the solution was to remain in the home and set emotional distance between my husband and myself.

I certainly recommend physical distance when a spouse and/or children have been or could be harmed from physical abuse. This type of boundary can provide time for healing as well as provide safety for the abused victims.

Sometimes we need a third person to help us feel more comfortable about setting boundaries or being truthful about how we feel. My initial therapist was the third person when I confronted my husband about certain feelings that I had and were afraid to express them to him alone. My therapist gave me the needed support to express my thoughts and my feelings.

Issues and concerns in relationships generally require both individuals working diligently over a period of time to solve a conflict. The issue probably did not occur overnight and therefore a solution will not be found overnight.

Remember if boundaries were never established or have been broken then it will require time for both partners to feel comfortable in setting boundaries and respecting the boundaries of each other.

## Establishing Boundaries for Me

I have basically lived my adult life without any set boundaries. When someone said something hurtful, I just filed it away in my invisible filing cabinet inside my heart and locked the door. When my husband would humiliate me in public, I added those insults to my filing cabinet. There were many times when I wanted to say how I really felt about an issue, but instead I said what I thought the other person wanted to hear. I filed those unhappy memories in by filing cabinet as well as the abuse I suffered as a child that I never talked about.

Then one day something happened that caused my invisible filing cabinet to explode. All the anger that I had filed away for so many years resulted in major depression and my not wanting to deal with life. I felt it was easier to commit suicide than to have to start revealing to people the real me that had been hiding inside for so long. By this time, I was not even sure if I knew who the real me was anymore.

My therapist gave me some information on setting boundaries. Boundary setting was not explained during the marriage vows, and I truly had only learned of boundary setting while conducting research for this book. So therefore I had a lot to learn.

For so many years, I have tolerated other people making decisions for me that I disagreed with. I did not allow myself to speak my opinion when asked, and I allowed myself to be controlled to the point of fearing the consequences if I did something my spouse would not approve of when he found out.

Lack of boundaries had left me with an angry, unforgiving spirit. I was angry at myself for tolerating the abuse and angry at others for abusing me. It became quite clear that I had to start setting boundaries if I was going to survive this bout of depression.

My first priority was setting boundaries for myself. In order to accomplish this, I had to focus on what I wanted instead of what others wanted. This may sound a little selfish, but I know from years of experience that putting my feelings aside to focus on the feelings of others has been nonproductive and damaging to me emotionally.

After years of denying myself, I really had to spend some time trying to figure out what I wanted in life. What are my dreams and desires? I must admit that I am still discovering who I am. It is not an easy process.

Although the self-discovery process is difficult, it will allow me to determine what I will tolerate and what I will not tolerate. I am learning to say 'no' to people even when their response is one of dissatisfaction. It is better for others to be temporarily unhappy than for me to regress back into a state of major depression.

Perhaps one of the greatest achievements for me during this process is realizing that I only have control over me. I can not control someone else's response to a situation. Another person's response is not something that I need to take ownership of. I only need to be responsible for me.

## Establishing Boundaries for Others

As a PTSD Veteran spouse, it is easy to feel that boundaries are worthless in your relationship when your husband suffers from PTSD. This is a fallacy. Whether or not your husband suffers from PTSD does not mean that you have to tolerate physical abuse, emotional abuse, or a controlling spouse. We feel that we have no control over ourselves as caregivers and therefore, we fail to set boundaries for ourselves. Remember we can not control our spouse, but we can control our own actions.

One boundary that my therapist helped me to set was the use of email to discuss issues between my spouse and myself. My husband has a controlling tone that makes me feel inferior and quite often words are said without any thought as to their effect on the other person. So I chose to ask my husband to respond to me only via email when he was upset with me about something, and I would in turn respond back to him via email. When you take the time to respond to an argument in a written format, it gives you time to think about what you are saying. It gives both participants time to think about what their partner wrote and then about the response he or she will send back. This boundary helped me a lot.

Noticed that I said I asked my husband to agree to this boundary. I can not demand anything of him. If he had responded by saying no he would not discuss matters with me through email, then I would have had to take matters one step further by explaining the consequences if he chose not to abide by a boundary that I was setting for myself. This boundary was to protect my heart and also help me to heal from emotional abuse.

So how do you set boundaries when a husband repeatedly comes home drunk with no consideration for you as his spouse? You simply tell him how it makes you feel when he comes home drunk. This can be tricky because we typically want to say things such as "you make me so mad" or "you have no respect for me". This is not expressing how you feel. You need to use the word "I". Instead, try "I feel angry and unappreciated when you come home drunk". "I feel that you are not respecting me as your wife." As in my case, it may take some time for you to get in contact with how you actually feel. Do not give up; it will get easier with time.

To establish a boundary with a husband who drinks too much and arrives home completely intoxicated, you simply tell him when he is sober that you will not continue to tolerate this behavior and if he chooses to come home again drunk that you will take the kids and spend the night with a family member, neighbor, or a friend and that you will let your host for the night know why you are there.

The boundary for a physically abusive spouse is difficult to say the least. You have to take into consideration your and your children's personal safety. The consequences of violating an established boundary in this situation can be difficult for the wife to enforce or could be life threatening. In a physically abusive situation, it is better to allow the abuser to calm down if you do not feel that there is the possibility of him injuring you to the point of death. The next day explain to your physically abusive husband that you will not tolerate being abused any longer and if he chooses to continue this behavior that you will take the kids and move out to a safe house or call the police and have him escorted from the premises. Then have all the locks changed immediately.

Notice that in the above situations you did not place a demand on your spouse but you gave him an option. If he chooses to continue his destructive behavior, he is well aware beforehand what the consequences will be. The breaking of boundaries must result in consequences for the boundary to be effective.

While establishing boundaries and consequences can be difficult, it becomes even more difficult to enforce the consequences once the boundary has been broken. It would be easier to let the children stay asleep in bed than go through with the consequence of spending the night elsewhere if he came home drunk one more time. It is important that you do exactly what you promised even if it would be easier to just ignore this latest episode. If you do not enforce the consequence, then the abusive husband will continue to be abusive.

The physically abusive spouse is normally very sorry for hitting you after it happens and well adept at making you believe that it was your fault that he chose to give you a black eye. Note that I said he chose. As the abused spouse, never believe the lie that it was your fault and do not tolerate being physically abused. If you allow it once, it says to your abusive husband that you will tolerate it again.

There are so many women who live in abusive situations out of fear that they can not make it on their own or trying to keep the family together for the sake of the children. Do not fool yourself into believing that the children are not aware of what is going on. The most important thing you can do is find a safe environment for you and your children. There are agencies opened 24 hours daily that will assist you. If you are in a physically abusive relationship, develop a safety plan. Have a friend or family member who is aware of your situation and are willing for you and the children to use their home as temporary shelter if you have to flee in the middle of the night.

The abusive husband must be reported to the police. Physical abuse is a crime. You simply can not allow him to not face the consequences of his actions. Remember he chose to hit you. You did not ask for it or deserve it. You have rights. If you need someone to be a support advocate for you through the process, then the various agencies established to handle domestic abuse cases can offer the support that you will need.

## Dealing with Enforcing the Consequences

You now know what you will and will not tolerate. You have set boundaries for yourself. You also are expressing to your spouse how his actions make you feel, and you have set forth consequences if he chooses to be abusive.

Now you must enforce the consequences when the boundaries are broken. Quite often you will deal with a spouse who will first play on your sympathy by saying "I promise, I won't do it again. This is the last time". If that does not work, then he will try blaming you for his choosing to do what he wanted to do. The third aspect is he will become irate when he realizes that this time you are not backing down. He now realizes that he is not dealing with the same person that tolerated his abuse in the past.

It can be extremely difficult to stand your ground, but it is absolutely essential that you do not back down. In the past, you never had boundaries so you just accepted whatever he chose to dish out to you. However, now you know that you have options and that you deserve to be treated with respect in the relationship, but it would be so much easier to go back to what is comfortable and familiar even if it ends up hurting you in the end. At least there will be peace for a short season.

After being sexually abused as a child, I never thought even as an adult that I had the right to set boundaries and enforce consequences if the boundaries were broken. I basically wanted other peoples' approval and I needed someone to protect me and love me – two things that were taken from me when the perpetrator chose to abuse me. Therefore, it was always easier to stay with what was comfortable and familiar because that provided some sense of safety to me.

However, after nineteen months of therapy with two different therapists and seventeen months of seeing a psychiatrist, I now realize that I am an independent woman capable of standing alone if I have to. If my spouse chooses to violate the boundaries I have set for myself, then I am gaining confidence that I do not have to stay and accept his disrespect of me just because it is comfortable. This mindset definitely did not happen overnight, and I realize that I still have much to learn about myself.

Enforcing the consequences is the hardest part. You must be somewhat comfortable with who you are as a person and you will need a strong friend or support group that will give you the strength to not give up.

As I mentioned previously, many spouses stay in marriages without boundaries out of fear. It is this fear of not knowing what will happen to them that keeps them in bondage. Marriage is not about one person doing as he or she chooses and the other person just has to deal with the abuse. Marriage is about two people respecting each other's boundaries and allowing each other the freedom to grow as an individual.

# How to Survive with a PTSD Spouse

PTSD is not an illness that you endure for a season and then it vanishes to never resurface again. If only it was that simple. PTSD is a daily part of life better known as a life of the unknown. You never know what symptom is going to greet you each day as you interact with your PTSD Veteran husband. So how do you survive and maintain your sanity. One step at a time – one moment at a time.

There will be many days when you will wish you had the courage to walk out the door and never look back, but on his good days you gather a sense of false hope that perhaps things will get better. The symptoms might improve with the proper treatment, but the symptoms will always exist to some degree.

So how do you survive if you choose to stay in such a volatile relationship? You may assume the role of caregiver, family protector, family mediator, financial supporter, sole children disciplinarian, and the list goes own. Your plate can become so full of caring for everyone and everything else that your needs get pushed so far down on the list until eventually they are not part of the list anymore. I know this to be fact, because it happened to me. Then one day when the kids were gone, I began to realize that I did not know who I was anymore. My life had become my husband's life, my daughter's life, and my son's life. I literally had no life without them. My function in life was to be sure that their lives went as smoothly as possible.

As I mentioned earlier, my son asked me recently why I never had friends when he was growing up. I thought that friends would have been a hindrance to me fulfilling my role as wife and mother. After all, I had a husband and two children who needed me why did I need friends. The truth of the matter is, it never occurred to me that I did not have friends during my children's years at home. It just never occurred to me that perhaps I needed a friend.

Women have an inner need for closeness that only female friends can supply. We need someone who will listen when we need to vent our frustrations and not try to fix the situation. We need someone that we can spend time talking to, sharing our secrets with, and dreaming about the future; we need someone that we can call just to talk when it seems that life has turned upside down. While men will listen, their first instinct is to offer a way to fix the problem. So in essence, men listen to provide a solution to the problem when sometimes we just want to talk.

As the spouse of a PTSD Veteran, it is more important than ever that you join or develop a support group of ladies that are in a similar situation as yourself. Only women with the same issues as you can support you. They can truly understand PTSD because they live with it daily as well.

It was in a support group of spouses that I realized that the symptoms displayed by my husband were not only peculiar to him but were being experienced by many other Veterans. It was a relief to know that I was not alone – that there were other wives just like me trying to understand

PTSD and survive in a life that we did not ask for but we had inherited by virtue of the fact our husbands had endured the traumas of war.

For so long, I never thought anyone else would understand what I was going through; and quite frankly, if that was all life had for me then I was not sure that remaining in such a painful state of living was something that I wanted to do.

If you are not familiar with any support groups, then I have listed numerous websites at the end of the book that will offer you some assistance. Some women prefer face to face support groups while other ladies prefer to remain anonymous in online support groups. If you prefer face to face support groups and you know at least one other lady who lives near you with a PTSD spouse, then the two of you can meet and support each other. When you are considering a support group, please keep in mind that PTSD is an illness that can result from any traumatic event, not just war.

Educate yourself on PTSD. Unfortunately, I lived for fourteen years not knowing that my husband had PTSD. He was not aware either. He was finally diagnosed when he retired from the Army. Once I found out he had the illness, I spent numerous hours reading as much as possible about the illness. The national PTSD Veterans Administration website offers a tremendous amount of information regarding the illness.

However, while there is an abundance of information regarding the Veteran, there is little to no information about the effects of PTSD regarding the spouse and family members of the Veteran. It would appear from the information that I read that PTSD only affects the Veteran. After nineteen years, I emphatically know that PTSD affects the spouse and the children as well. It has resulted in increased divorce rates, domestic abuse and an increased possibility of depression in the spouse and the children as well. The tentacles of PTSD can and do stretch throughout the Veteran's family.

The next step is to educate your children about PTSD. Do not assume that they do not notice that Dad is angry all the time or that he does not seem to want to be around them or that the two of you constantly argue. Children are quite perceptive even at an early age. If the Veteran is not willing to discuss PTSD with the children, then it becomes the spouse's responsibility.

Educating your children becomes a continuous process as they grow. Never think your two year old is too young for you to start explaining PTSD to him or her. Of course, a two year old can not comprehend the same information as a teenager so make your information age appropriate. This will help your children to better understand that their Dad's behavior is not their fault which is a common thought process for children. As a mother, I wish I had been able to better help my kids with understanding PTSD when they were growing up, but unfortunately, I had heard very little about PTSD until 2004 when my husband was diagnosed.

PTSD symptoms can result in many forms of responses such as isolation, emotional numbing, anger, depression, physical abuse, emotional abuse and mental abuse just to name some of the many symptoms. My problem as the spouse is that I personalized my husband's different mood swings. I always felt that it was my fault. I tried to make things better, but in my attempts to help, I quite often made things worse for myself. My mistake was internalizing and making my husband's PTSD symptoms my problem.

After dealing with severe depression, I now realize that his issues belong to him, and I do not own them. Therefore, we introduce boundaries into relationships to protect both individuals involved. If your PTSD spouse chooses to isolate himself, then that is his choice. You should not try to pull him out of his shell but give him time and space. During his periods of isolation, go do something that you enjoy. Do not worry about him. He will be fine. He just needs to be alone. If he is angry and wants to argue with you, simply tell him that you are leaving the room and will discuss the issue with him when he has calmed down.

Spouses tolerate many things from their PTSD husband. However, I am learning that much of what we tolerate is our own fault. Our PTSD husbands can be described by those on the outside of the four walls we call home as kind, loving, gentle, never gets angry, etc. Sometimes we as the spouse wonder who they are talking about. The person we live with is the total opposite which leads me to believe that if the PTSD Veteran can control his behavior in public then he can better control his behavior at home. It is up to us as the spouse to set limits on what we will and will not tolerate. The key is we must have consequences established if a boundary is broken, and we must be willing to enforce it. Otherwise boundaries are pointless.

As I have mentioned earlier, physical abuse should never be tolerated. There are numerous agencies which you can go to get help. You do not and should not stay in a physically abusive relationship. Your husband has no right to hit you or intimidate you in any way. It is a crime.

If you are in a physically abusive relationship and you are afraid to leave then develop an escape plan for yourself and your children in case the violence escalates to the point where you fear for your life and/or your children's lives. The PTSD Veteran wants you to believe that you can not survive without him, but you can. In many cases, women who have left their abusive husbands have gone on to become independent and happy women. They found the self confidence that their husband had taken from them.

Purchase a cell phone and hide it in a room that you can lock yourself in if your spouse becomes abusive. Dial 911 and let them hear the abusive language from your partner. They can locate you and send the police to escort the abusive husband to spend a night in the comfort of the city or county jail.

Develop a plan that if you have to leave suddenly you have access to money and a safe place to stay such as with a friend. It is important that you save money in order to sustain yourself and your children for a few days. Needless to say this information must be kept secretive from your husband unless you and he already have separate accounts.

Physical abuse is one of the primary reasons for leaving a spouse. The other which is less evident is emotional or mental abuse that has occurred over a long period of time. This develops into an element of control. In order for the husband to feel secure in the relationship, he feels that he must be in control of you and everything else. The question is does the controlled spouse stay because of love or fear. Can love exist when a person is controlled?

Emotional and mental abuse quite often leaves the wife in deep depression, suicidal, and fearful of her husband. Depending on the level of emotional and mental abuse, it can be better for the spouse to separate herself from the controlling partner. There may come a point where your emotional and mental stability are in question if you remain with your PTSD spouse. Instead of living a life in and out of severe depression, perhaps you should consider separation. Your health is worth more than a marriage that results in your emotional and mental instability.

All of the items listed above will help you as the spouse to reemerge. That is the most important aspect of this process is that 'you' began to realize that you are an important person in this relationship. You are a person with hopes, desires, and dreams of your own.

After 19 years of dealing with PTSD, I am finally learning that I am important as a person and as a woman. The things I tolerated in the past, I will not tolerate in the future. I have a life of my own to live. I will not take ownership of my husband's PTSD symptoms anymore. They belong solely to him.

Some may view this as selfish and that is their prerogative. However, they are probably not married to a PTSD spouse.

First and foremost, you can not lose your awareness of who you are. You have dreams. Pursue them. You have a life to live, and it should not be consumed by your attempt to avoid the next PTSD symptom that your husband exhibits. Believe me you can not prevent the symptoms because they seem to strike when you least expect them. I made the mistake of trying to prevent the symptoms from occurring. Two major bouts of depression and many suicidal thoughts later, I realized that I have no control over his symptoms. They belong to him. I only have control over me – my response and my actions.

After 19 years, I realize that I need friends and activities that I enjoy without my spouse. I enjoy spending a couple of hours reading and drinking coffee at the nearest coffee shop. I enjoy exercising and taking long walks. I also enjoy meeting a friend for lunch or dinner. Find something that you enjoy, and do it. You might enjoy gardening, spending time with friends, crafts, piano, volunteering, etc. The most important thing is that you do what makes you happy. Do those things that bring a smile to your face and make you feel good about yourself.

If you are going to survive in a world of PTSD, you must make **'you'** a priority,

Life isn't about waiting
for the storm to pass,
It's about learning to dance in the rain.

-author unknown

# Resources and Forums

If you or someone you love has PTSD, it is imperative that you educate yourself about this disorder so that you can better deal with your own symptoms or the symptoms of the person who has PTSD. This list contains websites that offer information on PTSD and also forums which will allow you to interact completely anonymously with other individuals who are experiencing the same difficulties that you are dealing with. I encourage you to take the time to investigate the information that is available for you.

http://health.groups.yahoo.com/group/vetwives/#ans

www.pmim.org

www.dcoe.health.mil/default.aspx

//health.groups.yahoo.com/group/SupportforPTSD

//home.comcast.net/~ptsdfamilies

www.bu.edu/bostonia/Spring09/gulf-war

www.ncptsd.va.gov

www.ptsdalliance.org

www.gulfweb.org

www.4militaryfamilies.com/articles/mentalhealth

www.sanctuaryweb.com/Documents/Caring for Caregi.pdf

www.peoplepreventsuicide.org/contamination_ptsd.php

www.theawarenesscenter.org/help.html

www.mayo-clinic.com

www.womanabuseprevention.com/html/trauma_post-traumatic_stress_.html

www.familyofavet.com/secondary_ptsd.html

www.vietnow.compagesptsd/ptsdeggshells.htm

www.ptsdforum.org/archive/index.php/t-5612.html

www.missfoundation.org/pro/articles/VicariousTrauma.pdf

www.aa.org

www.griefshare.org

www.divorcecare.org

www.dc4k.org

www.caregiver.com

# Suggested Readings

Batttlefield of the Mind
by Joyce Meyers

Boundaries – When to Say Yes How to Say No to Take Control of Your Life
by Dr. Henry Cloud and Dr. John Townsend

Boundaries in Marriage – Understanding the Choices that Make or Break Loving Relationships
by Dr. Henry Cloud and Dr. John Townsend

Praying Through the Deeper Issues of Marriage
by Stormie Omartian

Recovering From the War – A Woman's Guide to Helping Your Vietnam Vet, Your Family, and Yourself
by Patience H. C. Mason

The Wounded Woman – Hope and Healing for Those Who Hurt
By Dr. Steve Stephens and Pam Vredevelt

<u>Thrive, don't simply Survive</u> – Passionately Live the Life You Didn't Plan
by Karol Ladd

<u>Vietnam Wives</u> – Facing the Challenges of Life with Veterans Suffering Post-Traumatic Stress
by Aphrodite Matsakis, Ph.D.

<u>When the War is Over… A New One Begins</u> – Rebuilding Relationships after Trauma
by Chuck Dean and Bette Nordberg

# Endnotes

1.  National Center for PTSD
    http://www.ncptsd.va.gov/ncmain/fact_shts/fs_what_is_ptsd.html 3/13/2009

2.  Ibid
3.  Ibid
4.  Hummert, Heather A., Family of a Vet: Helping Children Understand PTSD
    http://www.familyofavet.com/helping_children_understand_PTSD.html